The
Type 1 Life

A Road Map for Parents of Children with Newly Diagnosed Type 1 Diabetes

Cover by Jess Creatives
Edited by Jodi Brandon Editorial

For more information, visit www.thetype1life.com.

ISBN: 978-0-692-07714-6
Library of Congress Control Number: 2018902914

Disclaimer: The information provided within is for general informational purposes only. The author has made every effort to include information up-to-date and correct, but there are no representations or warranties, express or implied, about the completeness, accuracy, reliability, suitability, or availability with respect to the information, products, services, or related graphics contained within. Any use of this information is at your own risk.

To my mom, dad, and sister: thank you for continuously going the extra mile for me over the last 27 years.

Table of Contents

Preface

...

When your child was diagnosed, the doctors had plenty of medical information to share with you. You learned how to handle low blood sugars, count carbohydrates, and give insulin. But, maybe your child's doctor didn't give you information about the day-to-day life as a child with Type 1 diabetes—like how to tell your child's classmates about Type 1 diabetes or how to handle sleepovers.

I had a conversation with a doctor once about some struggles I was having, and she said, "I get it! Well, actually, I don't." She knew what I was talking about because she talks to patients with Type 1 diabetes all day. But, she knows she doesn't **truly** understand the struggles, because she doesn't have Type 1 diabetes herself.

I've had Type 1 diabetes for 24 years, so it's second nature to me, but there are some things I wish I could've changed. My hope is that this book will provide some perspective on how to handle day-to-day life with a child who has Type 1 diabetes. I'm writing this guide for you, with the hope that it gives you insight and peace of mind.

In this book, you'll find many of my own experiences sprinkled in, as well as stories from other individuals with Type 1 diabetes, to give you some real-life examples. Type 1 diabetes can be messy, much like the cover of this book depicts. Every child and every family are different, so your child might not experience the same things and your family might handle things differently.

A Type 1 diagnosis can be scary and overwhelming for you and for your child, but in time, you'll find your groove and find that it's manageable. Having diabetes over the last 24 years has not held me back from traveling, getting married, or running my own business. Thanks to modern medicine, Type 1 diabetes is not a death sentence.

The content in this book is not meant to be or replace medical advice. Always listen to your doctor's instructions when it comes to your child's health.

Chapter 1
A New Normal

...

A Barbie corvette.

That's the only thing I remember about the time I spent in the hospital after being diagnosed with Type 1 diabetes. I was barely three years old, and it was July 4, 1993. My parents, on the other hand, remember feeling completely overwhelmed—similar to what you may be feeling.

As odd as it may sound, I'm grateful that I was diagnosed as a three-year-old. I don't remember a life without insulin injections. I didn't have to switch from regular soda to diet soda. I don't have a before and after.

Because I was so young, I couldn't exactly say *glucometer*. Early on, my parents named my glucometer George. I don't know if they intended for the name to stick, but up until I left for college, our entire family called it George. Naming the glucometer George made things a little less scary for me as a child and a little easier to talk about in public places. "Did you grab George?" they would ask as we headed out the door. "Have you checked George?" they would ask before we'd start eating dinner at a restaurant.

As I'm writing this, I've had diabetes for 24 years, but it feels like I was born with diabetes. That's 24 years of insulin shots, counting calories and carbs, eating honey and glucose tabs, feeling nauseous from high blood sugars, and countless doctor appointments. No "off" switch, no remission, no breaks. And as much as I try to stay in control, there is still the very real possibility of developing complications down the road.

Having diabetes has always affected my self-image and self-esteem, but the hardest part of living with Type 1 diabetes is that it has affected, and will always affect, my family and our day-to-day lifestyle. Type 1 diabetes is a team effort, and there's guilt that comes with it, knowing I'm adding extra stress to others' lives. Not to mention, as a diabetic, we're always thinking about what could go wrong next week, next year, or in 10 years—without trying to totally lose hope. It's a stress that only other individuals with Type 1 diabetes understand.

The hardest part of living with Type 1 diabetes is that it has affected, and will always affect, my family and our day-to-day lifestyle.

Why Me?

"Why me?"

Depending on your child's age, this may be a question they've already asked, or one they'll ask in a few years. In fact, they may ask it several times as they're growing up. Unfortunately, there's no great answer.

It's important to remind your child that it's not their fault, and it's not your fault. My family has a strong faith background, so my parents believed that God wasn't testing us, but that God knew we would be strong and smart enough to handle it.

I still believe this, and I believe that anyone growing up with Type 1 diabetes will be stronger, smarter, and more independent. While I still get frustrated with diabetes from time to time, I stopped asking, "Why me?" when I came to accept my condition. Acceptance came with age and with more independence in my care.

I still vaguely remember giving myself my first insulin shot as a second grader at our kitchen table. Up until that point, my parents had always been the ones to check my blood sugar and give me my shots. I have no idea why I was so eager to jab myself with a needle, but thus began my journey into becoming more independent.

As scary as it may be, encouraging this independence is important—at whatever age you find is appropriate. Nothing about Type 1 diabetes is cookie-cutter, and how you handle each situation will depend on your child. Someday, your child will live on their own. They need to be fully capable of not only checking their own blood sugar and giving their own insulin shots, but also making their own doctor's appointments and calling their insurance provider.

Nat Strand won *The Amazing Race*, Crystal Bowersox almost won *American Idol*, and Nick Jonas is a successful singer and actor in Hollywood. It's safe to assume these individuals are independently managing their Type 1 diabetes without a parent holding their hand. While it probably didn't happen overnight, their parents had to, at some point, foster this spirit of independence in their children.

Educating Others

After your child's diagnosis, you'll need to tell people about their diabetes. With social media, it's easy to tell several people at once, so you can opt to do this to save time. There are some people who you'll want to have more in-depth conversations with, though, especially those who will be around your child often—neighbors, babysitters, church group leaders, and parents of friends, for example.

Part of "owning" their diagnosis involves your child being

able to openly share about it when necessary. Maybe it's not the first thing your child brings up in a conversation, but there's no need to be embarrassed or ashamed of having Type 1 diabetes.

When I had to start taking shots before lunch in grade school, my parents and I decided it was best to only tell a few of my closest friends. I had been at this school for two and a half years, so everyone knew I had Type 1 diabetes. This new information wasn't something that everyone needed to know, though, because it didn't affect them. Discuss with your child who they feel comfortable telling about their diagnosis. It might be beneficial to meet with their friends, and their friends' parents, so everyone knows why this happened and how to handle things moving forward.

These conversations will also involve describing the distinction between Type 1 and Type 2 diabetes. It's not uncommon for people to reference diabetes and not make the distinction between Type 1 and Type 2. Type 1 diabetes is an autoimmune disease, whereas Type 2 diabetes is usually caused by lifestyle factors or genetics. Type 1 diabetics have a pancreas that no longer produces any insulin, so they will always need to take insulin to stay alive (or at least until there is a cure). Type 2 diabetics have a pancreas that may produce some insulin, but not enough. Type 2 diabetics can usually control their diabetes with exercise, diet, and oral medications (but may need to eventually also start taking insulin). In my late

20s, I'm still having to describe the difference to people and explain that I didn't get diabetes from eating too much candy.

You may have people tell you random "cures" for your child's Type 1 diabetes. Among the more interesting "cure myths" I've heard: exercising more, doing a cleanse, taking cinnamon pills, drinking okra or cucumber water, and using essential oils. These unusual ideas come from people who are misinformed about the differences between Type 1 and Type 2 diabetes, and how the body works.

For people who might be around your child often, you may want to do some sort of informal training for them. When I was young, my mom created a booklet of diabetes information to give to teachers and babysitters. It folded horizontally, and each section had a tab with a title like low blood sugars, snacks, and glucagon treatment. It was small enough to hang on a refrigerator, and easy enough to flip to the right section when they needed to remember how much insulin to give me. You can download a template at www.thetype1life.com, to give to friends' parents, chaperones, neighbors, and any other adult who may need it.

Recognizing Patterns

Your child's doctor likely discussed this with you, but if not, it's important to keep track of your child's blood sugars in a physical log book, or on an app, and make notes with each blood sugar check or insulin dosage. At the end of each week or month, review this data. You might see that your weekly family pizza night is raising your child's blood sugar, or that their blood sugar runs higher on the days of basketball games. This is something you should continue to do as your child grows up, because patterns may change and new patterns may develop.

Thanks to modern technology, there are three types of smartphone apps that can benefit individuals with Type 1 diabetes: blood sugar logs, carbohydrate counters, and continuous glucose monitoring apps. Each category has variations, and more apps being developed every year, but I want to highlight some of the more popular types of apps to get you started.

Blood Sugar Logs

Growing up, I had to write down my blood sugars on paper, but now you can keep track of everything digitally. MySugr: Diabetes Tracker Log and Glucose Buddy Diabetes Tracker allow you to track blood sugar levels, record insulin intake, track carbs, and track any other miscellaneous info you want to track with regard to your child's health. Though both apps have free versions, you can pay a small fee per month for additional features.

There are glucometers available that also have a smartphone app: Accu-Chek® Aviva Connect, CONTOUR® NEXT ONE, Dario Smart Glucose Meter, One Drop | Chrome, and One-

Touch Verio Flex®, to name a few. Each of the meters connects with their app, and makes it easy to review blood sugars and share data. These glucometers and apps save you the trouble of having to remember to manually log your child's blood sugars.

Carbohydrate Counters

Whether you're eating out or at a family friend's house, your child will often be in situations in which you don't know the exact calorie or carbohydrate count of a particular food. Plenty of apps allow you to search nutrition facts for foods, but MyFitnessPal and CalorieKing are two that I recommend. Both apps also have the option to upgrade for additional features.

Continuous Glucose Monitor Apps

If your child has a continuous glucose monitor (also known as a CGM, which I'll talk about later in this book), there are a few apps that you can download to use in conjunction with the CGM. To start, Dexcom has an iPhone app to act as the CGM receiver. You can also download apps like Sugarmate to enable more notifications or Diabits to get blood sugar predictions based on your child's activity. Neither of these apps has the option to upgrade.

***

A new diagnosis is stressful because everything feels overwhelming. There are so many new things to remember and numbers to track. Unfortunately, the bad news is that diabetes can be unpredictable. Your child might do the same things two days in a row and get different results. The good news is, despite the unpredictability, you will hopefully and eventually start to notice patterns.

To help identify patterns, set a consistent schedule. This schedule may not be possible all of the time with school activities and traveling, but adhering to a some type of schedule reduces the number of variables in what feels like a never-ending science experiment called Type 1 diabetes. Without a consistent schedule, it'll be harder to determine which specific foods or activities are causing any high or low blood sugars.

For example, one of the patterns that my parents noticed around junior high is that the weather affects my blood sugars. It sounds silly, and I've never had a doctor who believes me, but it rings true to this day. Day-to-day weather doesn't really affect me (unless it's 110 degrees outside), but the seasons changing wreaks havoc. Every year, the one- or two-week transition from fall to winter, and from spring to summer, causes my blood sugars to go haywire.

My parents also noticed a very specific symptom that signaled a low blood sugar: The circles under my eyes would darken. This is not something that doctors said would happen or is even listed as a common symptom of Type 1 diabetics. My parents also noticed I would become really irritable, which also signaled that I was probably low. (Maybe not every time: Sometimes I was just being a teenager.) Your child may have their own unusual symptoms as well.

It's Just a Check

Part of the everyday—more like, all day, everyday—routine for individuals with Type 1 diabetes is checking our blood sugar. At a minimum, we're supposed to check our blood sugars four times per day. Doctors typically recommend checking before each meal, and before going to sleep.

Depending on the age of your child, you may need to check their blood sugar for them, or simply help them. As your child gets older, they will need to start claiming more responsibility for their own blood sugars. You know your child best, but middle school is when I recommend they be able to start handling most of their own blood sugar checks, insulin injections, and calorie counting.

Every person has their own preferences for checking blood sugars. Some only use certain fingers for the test. (I can't use my index finger or thumbs, for example.) Some use no fingers at all, and decide to use their arms for the test. Everyone tends to develop a preference for a certain glucometer brand. (There is always the chance that your insurance provider will decide it likes another glucometer brand, and your child's preferred brand may not be covered any longer.)

When it comes to checking my blood sugar consistently, I struggle—but not because it hurts or it's too time-consuming. I struggle because for so many years, this check was more like a pass/fail test. People use both the terms *check* and *test* when talking about this process with our glucometer. I've had to intentionally focus on changing my vocabulary to only call it a blood sugar check. Though it was never talked about in this way, my family's reactions to my blood sugar levels made it feel like a pass/fail test. A good blood sugar meant I was a good diabetic. A high or low blood sugar meant I was a bad diabetic—a bad person.

If we take this train of thought a step further, many people try not to even call someone with Type 1 diabetes a diabetic. I am not a diabetic wife, or a diabetic athlete, or a diabetic daughter. I am a wife, an athlete, a daughter—and I also happen to have Type 1 diabetes. For that reason, you'll notice that I tried to limit the use of the word *diabetic* in this book.

Whether you call it a check or a test doesn't matter all that much; what really matters is your reaction to your child's blood sugars. My parents never yelled at me or punished me for bad blood sugars, but it didn't go without an occasional disapproving look or a small lecture about needing better blood sugar control. It's a hard act to balance, and your child may need that reminder (like I did), because good control is necessary for good health.

I am a wife, an athlete, a daughter—and I also happen to have Type 1 diabetes.

Also be aware of your body language and comments if your child has a high blood sugar. They are not a good or bad diabetic, daughter, or son, because of their blood sugars.

A blood sugar is just a number, and your child is still a child. Be intentional about having conversations with them besides just constantly asking about their blood sugars. Make an effort to not have your first question always be about their current blood sugars.

In addition, there are a few things you can do in terms of positive reinforcement:

- Praise them for checking their blood sugar at all! In just one year, your child will probably check their blood sugar at least 1,500 times. It's not fun, it hurts, and it gets old—really fast. If they are checking as they should, applaud their diligence.
- Praise them when they make smart food choices. As a child, it's easy to want to beg for "regular" sweets or other snacks. If they make a smart food choice on their own, applaud their efforts to be responsible instead of indulgent.
- Praise them just for being themselves! Let them know that you see their struggles and that you know it's not fun or easy to have diabetes.

Action Steps

1. Create a list of who you want to tell about your child's diagnosis. Make a note of who should receive more in-depth training.

2. Decide how you will track your child's blood sugars and how often you will sit down to review the data.

Chapter 2
Doctors and Insurance

...

The door was closed, but I remember hearing his voice bellow loudly as he talked to the patient. It was obvious that the patient in the room was not managing their diabetes like they should.

After hearing this, I didn't want to go in—much less by myself.

My mom was with me, but since I was in middle school, she wanted me to start going into the exam room alone—to be more independent. Dr. Guthrie was my endocrinologist from the very start, and even with his big hugs, I always felt timid around him. He was a doctor who meant business, and he knew when you weren't doing what you were supposed to do. Dr. Guthrie was so good that we sometimes drove two hours just to see him for a half an hour.

As a child, I didn't fully understand how great a doctor he was, or even the importance of a great doctor. It didn't hit me until college, when I had to switch doctors. (Side note: Make sure your child lists you as a contact on any of their HIPAA release forms. More on this in Chapter 8.) For about six years, I struggled to find a decent endocrinologist. I ran into some doctors who weren't a great fit for me, for varying reasons:

- One told me I was healthy and beautiful when I asked about how to lose weight as a Type 1 diabetic.
- One seemed to have an anger problem.
- One didn't even look at my blood sugars, instead asked me how I was feeling, and wanted to adjust my insulin settings based on that alone.
- Another also didn't look at my blood sugars and spent the least amount of time with me of any other doctor I've visited.

If there's one thing my mom taught me, and something that I hope you teach your own children, it's that **you have to be your own best advocate.** We drove two hours because Dr. Guthrie was the best, and he was worth it. It's okay to challenge your child's doctor, or to go to two different doctors in a year.

One of the hardest parts of being an individual with diabetes is never feeling like you're doing enough. Especially as a teenager, when it feels like so many variables are out of your control, doctor appointments are not enjoyable because you are scrutinized and given a list of things to work on.

One of the hardest parts of being an individual with diabetes is never feeling like you're doing enough.

When my friend Ellie Hook, who has had Type 1 diabetes for 19 years, was in college, she went to an endocrinologist appointment in which her new doctor said, "Wow, you're working really hard to manage your disease. I see you check consistently, but your blood sugars are all over the board. As you know, that's totally normal for adolescents. We can make a modification here since you're trending high at this time." As a diabetic, it is very rare to actually have a doctor acknowledge our hard work and not throw blame. All individuals deserve this type of care from their doctors, but it's not always a reality.

What to Look For

You will be seeing your child's endocrinologist and diabetes care team regularly, so you want people you can fully trust with your child's health.

While I do reference endocrinologists in this book, many patients with Type 1 diabetes are instead seen by a nurse practitioner and a diabetes educator. In some offices, the endocrinologist is the primary provider of information, and your child will only see a diabetes educator or dietician on occasion. Other times, most of the diabetes care is carried out by a diabetes nurse specialist or nurse practitioner, under the care of an endocrinologist. Either route is fine, as long as you are happy with the standard of care.

Since you are likely reading this book sometime in the first few months or year of your child's diagnosis, don't be too picky. The hospital may have referred you to someone, and it's fine to stick with that doctor. In fact, you may love him or her! The following factors are things to keep in mind in the future, should you ever need a new doctor.

Availability

When you call to make an appointment, how booked is the doctor? Having to wait six months is not a good sign. You want to find some middle ground, say one to three months. If you can't see someone for six months, it likely means they are overbooked. When a doctor is overbooked, your appointment may start late, and you may feel rushed during the appointment. There are several things to cover in an appointment, so you want adequate time to discuss everything with your doctor. Also, ask the doctor if you can call with questions, or submit blood sugars between appointments. Most doctors want to see their patients every three to four months.

Changes

Thanks to research, we have so much information about how to handle diabetes through a variety of scenarios. With the help of technology, managing diabetes has become incredibly easier. But, even with research and technology, there are still hiccups in controlling blood sugars and being a healthy individual. Is your doctor open to trying new things, like new medicines or devices? I kept asking doctors for advice on losing weight, to no avail. Finally, when I asked a new doctor this same question, I was given a few options. My doctor didn't push these options on me, and she laid out the pros and cons of each.

Talking to Your Child

Does the doctor talk directly to your child? When I was first diagnosed at three years old, I have no idea if my doctor actually spoke to me (probably not). But, as I got older, he would speak directly to me with questions and tell me what changes he was making in my regimen. I was a shy little girl, so this often intimidated me. Looking back, this was his way of helping me take ownership of my diabetes.

Questions and Discussion

Your child's doctor should allow both of you to ask questions and address any issues. (If you ever feel an issue is urgent, call the doctor's office; do not wait until the next appointment.) In my experience, doctors who are overbooked and rushed usually want to do the bare minimum. As I've mentioned, many things affect blood sugars, so you need to discuss these with your child's doctor. Some things you might want to discuss at each appointment are:

- New symptoms or problems you've noticed (even if unrelated to diabetes).

- Any major changes that have occurred since your child's last visit.
- New medications that your child has started taking (even if unrelated to diabetes).
- Updates to family medical history.

Data

Since I mentioned it previously, you probably expected this to make the list: Doctors need to actually look at blood sugars. I used to have to write down all of my blood sugars in a log book and bring it to appointments, but now it's as easy as letting the doctor download your child's blood sugars from the glucometer. Once they've downloaded your glucometer, they can look at averages, patterns, before-meal levels, after-meal levels, and more. From there, they will make any necessary adjustments to insulin levels and ratios. (Some offices prefer if you download or send this data ahead of time, so be sure to ask for the doctor's preference if they don't mention it.)

Overall Health

Appointments will usually start with checking your child's height, weight, and blood pressure. The doctor should be asking about your child's overall health and be communicating with your child's other doctors. If there are any concerning reports or notes from other doctors, they will discuss it at your child's appointment. Also, endocrinologists generally check your child's reflexes and check their feet to make sure there aren't signs of neuropathy.

Blood Work

A few times each year, your child will need to have blood drawn and provide a urine sample. The best scenario is having the tests done a week before your appointment with the doctor (so they can review the results with you). Often, though, you will have blood work done after an appointment, and they will just call you with results. The doctor will look at a variety of things, but the one result talked about the most is the A1C. The A1C test shows the average blood sugar levels over the past three months. Based on those results, your child's doctor will make adjustments to their insulin and food ratios, if needed. (I always describe this to people without Type 1 diabetes as my diabetes GPA.)

Other Doctors

You'll most often visit an endocrinologist, because this is the doctor that assists in the actual management of your child's diabetes. For a child with diabetes, optimal health requires a team of doctors. Your child will need to visit these doctors regularly, if they aren't already.

Eye Doctor

People with diabetes who struggle with high blood sugars are at risk for damaged blood vessels in the retina, commonly referred to as diabetic retinopathy. It cannot be cured, only prevented with good blood sugar management. You'll want to be sure your child's blood sugars are in good control during the day of each eye exam so that results are accurate.

Dentist

People with diabetes are also at a higher risk for gum disease when blood sugars are not controlled. Regular visits to the dentist are important to keep teeth clean and to stay on top of any infections that may develop.

Podiatrist

Another common complication associated with Type 1 diabetes is neuropathy, because people with diabetes are prone to poor blood flow and nerve damage. It's unlikely your child will need to see a podiatrist until after puberty, unless the endocrinologist notices a problem. (I didn't see one until after college.)

Dealing with Insurance and Supply Companies

In addition to doctors, you'll also be interacting a lot with insurance companies and medical supply companies—especially if your child has an insulin pump or continuous glucose monitor (CGM).

I can't tell you the number of times that my insurance company sent me a letter announcing that it would no longer cover something that I use. I've had to change insulin brands, needles, and glucometers many times over the years. For me, and many others, the most frustrating part is that insurance often changes again, causing you to switch back, sometimes less than a year later.

Having to deal with insurance so often is part of why it's so important to have a great doctor. You want a doctor, or a doctor's staff, who is responsive and willing to send paperwork (sometimes repeatedly) to your insurance provider so you can get the supplies you need.

Here are a few quick tips for calling insurance or medical supply companies:

- Try to call first thing in the morning when representatives haven't been hounded all day.
- Take notes during your call.
- Get the name and number of the person with whom you spoke.
- If possible, get confirmation numbers for orders or claims submitted.

If (or when) your insurance won't cover a particular brand of insulin or device, you can try to petition them for an exception. You and your doctor will need to send a letter of medical necessity, explaining why you believe the company should cover your child's particular needs. This process can take weeks or even months.

Based on what insurance and medical companies have had me write before, your letter of medical necessity should include:

- A description of your child's condition.
- Any challenges your child experienced with different brands.
- Your child's personal medical history, especially any dangerous incidences .
- Rationale for why this device or brand is needed.
- Why your child would benefit from this particular device or brand.

You should also ask your doctor and insurance provider if there is anything else that needs included in the letter of necessity.

Switching Insurance Companies

Inevitably, you will likely switch insurance companies at least a few times in your life. There are a few details to specifically ask about when it comes to switching companies or plans:

- The deductible and out-of-pocket costs.
- Coverage for durable medical equipment (your pump and sensor).
- If durable medical equipment has a different coinsurance than other things.
- How/where pump supplies, prescriptions, test strips, and CGM supplies fit in their plan.
- Their drug/prescription formulary, as that will affect your cost on insulin.

Action Steps

1. If your child has other doctors they see regularly, call those doctors' offices and let them know about your child's diagnosis. It may be that they just make a note in your child's file, or they may want your child to come in for an appointment.

2. If it's not in the same place where you track your child's blood sugars, decide where you will write down any non-urgent questions to ask at your child's next appointment. You might consider having one notebook in which you write down questions for your doctor, notes from calls, etc.

Chapter 3
Insulin Pumps and Continuous Glucose Monitors

...

You may remember that we referred to my glucometer as George when I was growing up. It was George because it also started with a G like glucometer. Several years after getting my insulin pump in high school, my sister and I named that as well: Milly. (We decided on Milly because the company that makes my pump starts with an M.) The rest of my family doesn't refer to it as Milly, but both my husband and I do!

I remember seeing an insulin pump for the first time at Camp Discovery (which you'll learn about in Chapter 7). I was still in grade school at the time, so the doctors and education staff weren't getting too technical with us yet. I remember thinking that the few campers who did have an insulin pump had something "extra wrong" with them. (Clearly, I hadn't been fully educated on what an insulin pump was and why it was so beneficial to people with Type 1 diabetes.)

I didn't get my first insulin pump until I was a senior in high school, once the price had come down, and we had good insurance coverage. Not a single classmate teased me about my insulin pump. In fact, many of them thought it was really interesting. I lived in a rural area, so I had to miss about a week of school to travel to my doctor four hours away, get the insulin pump, and get the necessary training for it from my diabetes educator. Because I was gone for so long, and hadn't explicitly shared details, many of my classmates were worried and thought I had undergone surgery and was in the hospital all week.

The only exception was the junior high student who thought my insulin pump was an mp3 player, and asked why I got to bring my mp3 player to school and he didn't. Other than that, life continued as normal. An insulin pump can easily fit into pants pockets, so it's typically not too visible. Most of the time, if someone notices it, it's because they are either diabetic themselves or have a close family member who has an insulin pump.

Having an insulin pump is not cheap, but the convenience is so worth it. I've now had my insulin pump for 10 years, and it's hard to imagine going back to multiple daily injections. The pump has two main functions: boluses and basal rates. A bolus is taken with food, or to correct high blood sugars. A basal rate is background insulin, similar to how an IV slowly administers medicine, to keep blood sugar levels more consistent throughout the day. Some patients eventually choose to take a break from their insulin pump, though, because they don't want to stay tethered to a device forever.

There are a few reasons for you to consider getting an insulin pump for your child:

- Wearing an insulin pump means your child won't have to carry around a needle and bottle of insulin. When eating at a restaurant, your child wouldn't have to try to be discreet, or go to the restroom to take their insulin.
- Insulin pumps can deliver more accurate and specific insulin dosages. For example, with insulin injections, your child can take 12 units or, with an insulin pump, 12.7 units. Individuals can also use square or dual-wave boluses, which spread out the bolus over a specified amount of time.
- Individuals can obtain greater control of their blood sugars with varied basal rates. For example, for optimal blood sugar levels, my doctor and I have set six different basal rates throughout the day. One of the morning basal rates is lower, because I work out in the mornings, and it lessens the chance of my blood sugar going low.

While we're talking about insulin pumps, it's also important to briefly talk about continuous glucose monitors (CGMs), because they are often purchased and used together (though they don't have to be). Your doctor will likely discuss this with you, but if they haven't yet, a CGM is a small sensor inserted into the skin that continuously provides insight into glucose levels.

What's really great about having a CGM is that it sends updates to a receiver or your smartphone every few minutes, so you constantly know what your child's blood sugar levels are. It sounds a small alarm if your child's blood sugars are rapidly rising or falling, so you can be aware that they may need treatment soon. I use a Dexcom sensor, and I have the ability to send certain alerts to my husband's phone. Since I run my own business and work alone from my home, this extra alert feature provides some peace of mind for my husband and me.

Doctors are typically advocates of CGMs because you can really keep tighter control on blood sugars. I didn't get a CGM until a few years after college, when my doctor recommended it to improve my blood sugar control. It can also turn into a roundabout way for individuals to gamify Type 1 diabetes care. People post pictures of their daily graph on social media, bragging about how they were finally able to stay within a certain range for a certain amount of time.

Troubleshooting

As great as they are, insulin pumps don't come without their problems! I've definitely had my fair share of annoyances and had to figure out what to do with my insulin pump in different scenarios. Even though pumps come with a manual, and you will undergo training with your doctor before your child starts wearing it, here's some insight on troubleshooting common problems that come with an insulin pump:

One of the first things to note is that your child needs to rotate their pump site. The pump reservoir and site need to be changed every two to three days. You want to be sure to rotate the location of their site. Just like with insulin shots, tissue can build up under the skin if a site is in the same spot too often. I try to do a rotation, like left side of the stomach, right side of the stomach, left leg, right leg, and so on. If you don't rotate often enough, your child may develop small lumps, and your child's insulin won't absorb properly.

As can any technology, pumps can sometimes quit at the most inopportune times. (For me, one of those times was during my husband's and my move into our first house!) There's no warning; the pump simply starts buzzing or beeping, and displays an error message. Sometimes it's an error message to do with the reservoir, and other times the screen freezes and the pump stops completely.

If your child's insulin pump goes on the fritz, and you need to get a new one, there are two things to do. First, call your insulin pump company and report the issue. They'll ask you a few questions to confirm that it does need to be replaced. Because these devices administer life-saving medicine, the company will prioritize replacement shipping, and can usually get a new insulin pump to you within a day or two. Depending on your insurance coverage and the warranty on the pump, you may need to pay for part of the replacement. After that step, call your child's doctor.

Usually, the doctor will call in a prescription for a long-acting insulin for your child to take until their insulin pump arrives. You'll need to go to the pharmacy to get this new insulin, as well as some needles if you don't have any on hand. It's easy to keep some spare needles around, but because insulin has a short shelf life, it doesn't financially make sense to keep it on hand at all times. (You can also buy NPH insulin at the pharmacy without a prescription.)

Again, these insulin pump malfunctions aren't too common and, though annoying, can be easily handled.

The Emotional Toll of Insulin Pumps

Insulin pumps can come with their occasional technical problems, as well as an emotional and mental toll. Even after being on an insulin pump for 10 years, though, the downsides are outweighed by the benefit of being on a insulin pump.

As diabetic children, we are usually already the odd man out. Wearing a device 24/7 has the potential to add fuel to that fire. Luckily, this wasn't the case for me. My sister didn't like the idea of me getting an insulin pump in high school for this very reason: It made my invisible disease more visible. Before your child gets an insulin pump, it's a good idea to have them practice answering "What is that?" and other questions.

Getting an insulin pump also requires an internal adjustment period. Though it's not painful, it is a new experience to be attached or tethered to a device at all times. Through trial and error, they'll figure out how to wear their pump when sleeping, while playing sports, and when wearing clothes without pockets, and what to do at special occasions like a wedding. It should only take a few times for the tubing to catch on a doorknob and pull out the pump site for your child to learn to hide the excess tubing in their pocket! Because insulin pumps are so popular now, there are actually plenty of insulin pump accessories: covers, pouches, cases, and more.

At the end of the day, there's no right or wrong way to for your children to feel about their insulin pump—and their feelings about it might change. Over time, all the data intake and the site changes may be too much, and they'll want to take a break from it.

Diabetic Alert Dogs

In addition to CGMs, many people with diabetes are beginning to utilize diabetic alert dogs. Lauren Burke was diagnosed with Type 1 diabetes when she was 12 years old. A few years later, her endocrinologist told her about diabetic alert dogs, but most organizations wouldn't place an alert dog with someone younger than 18. It wasn't until Lauren got to college that she started researching and jumping through all the hoops to try to get her own diabetic alert dog.

After Lauren graduated from college, she was placed with her current alert dog, Ricki. Ricki alerts Lauren to high blood sugars, low blood sugars, and blood sugar changes greater than 10%. Lauren finds that Ricki beats her Dexcom G6 sensor by 20+ minutes every time. Ricki alerts in real time: She smells the chemical changes in Lauren's body as they are happening, whereas CGMs wait for the blood from your core to get into your interstitial fluid.

Lauren still wears her CGM religiously, because there is so much an alert dog doesn't tell you, nor are they perfect animals. For example, an alert dog can't catch your blood sugars drifting up at 2 a.m. if it's not taking you out of your normal blood sugar range. And, Lauren has learned not to expect night alerts if she and Ricki had an overly active day.

It seems like an incredible thing (you can take your dog anywhere!), but you have to remember your child is not taking their dog *anywhere*—they're taking their dog *everywhere*. Everywhere your child goes, people may point and stare. You'll have to tell people every day to not distract the dog, because the dog is working. You have to patiently educate people. Very few people assume a dog is an alert dog, and if they do, they often assume you're blind. Every day, people assume Lauren is training her dog, when in reality they've been together for more than three years.

According to Lauren, an alert dog won't make your job as a Type 1 diabetic much easier. A well-trained dog will be taught to never give up, and if their human doesn't act to correct an out-of-range blood sugar, the dog should go to alert more people. You can't cheat or turn the alarms off on a dog! Lauren says having a dog constantly alert you for several hours can be a lot to mentally and emotionally handle. There have been times when Lauren has gotten frustrated with her own dog, because she's already corrected her high blood sugar, but her blood sugar is not budging--and Ricki continues to alert. But you can't get mad at the dog, because they're doing their job, and this is what you want and need them to do.

If you are interested in potentially getting a diabetic alert dog, Assistance Dogs International (ADI) is the global accrediting body of service animals. ADI holds nonprofits to high standards in an effort to make sure they take good care of the consumers. ADI also partners with governments across the globe to standardize service animals and their public access rights. If your alert dog is not from an ADI-accredited organization, it can make traveling out of the country more difficult. (Each country has different laws and public access standards, so make sure to do your research before you plan your trip!)

Good organizations put in a lot of time and effort to place

people with the right dog. For example, Early Alert Canines spends a whole day with each client working with each dog to make sure an appropriate match is made. Finding the right match is important, and each dog should match their human partner's energy level and lifestyle. A lazy, low-key dog wouldn't be a good match for an active, on-the-go triathlete, for example, and an energetic, playful dog wouldn't be a good match for a household with very young children or caring for an elderly relative.

Action Steps

1. Talk to your child's doctor about the potential of getting an insulin pump or continuous glucose monitor (CGM). Ask about the different options that are available for each.

2. Call your insurance provider to see if an insulin pump or continuous glucose monitor would be covered under your plan. You may want to ask if coverage would be different for different brands.

Chapter 4
Family and Support Systems

...

My whole family loved volleyball. Both my sister and I played school and club volleyball while we were in high school. Club volleyball takes place outside of the regular school-sponsored volleyball season, and teams are formed with players from various geographic areas. The teams meet in a central location for practice, and then travel to big tournaments, sometimes in large cities and often in neighboring states. It was a lot of fun for our family of volleyball fanatics!

Club volleyball was also pretty pricey. Team members' families were responsible for paying for uniforms as well as travel-related costs (gas, hotels, food, etc.) to go to tournaments. I distinctly remember driving home with my parents after practice one night when they started talking about money, not knowing I was actively listening. Both of my parents had good jobs with good insurance, but not all of my diabetes supplies were fully covered. Upon hearing their conversation,

I told them I would quit club volleyball, and I didn't finish the season.

I quit out of guilt. I felt guilty that they were spending so much money, not just on club volleyball, but for all of my diabetes supplies, food, and doctors' appointments. Diabetes is not cheap.

Your child may eventually carry around a similar guilt. Doctors don't tell you about the mental and emotional toll that this disease can take on you, your child, and your family. My parents were incredibly caring and never meant to intentionally make me feel guilty. In fact, they didn't even know about this guilt that I had, because I didn't know how to tell them.

It's important to have open conversations with your child about how they are feeling, and what they might be struggling with as a child with Type 1 diabetes. If it's not guilt that your child feels, it may be shame, bitterness, or any number of other emotions. Your child having open communication with someone—whether it's you, an aunt or uncle, a schoolteacher, or a neighbor—is always important. Depending on the severity of these emotions, you may need to consider having them also visit with a counselor.

Your child's Type 1 diabetes is not a reason to limit them from school or community activities. Trying to juggle the club volleyball schedule and activity level was not easy on my blood sugars, but my parents didn't let that stop me. Your child can still stay at a friend's house overnight for a sleepover; it will just take **Your child's Type 1 diabetes is not a reason to limit them from school or community activities.** a little forethought. Your child can still go on school trips; it will just require preparing and training the chaperones.

It's important that your child fully understand the gravity of their diagnosis and that they don't ignore symptoms or handle their care inappropriately. Because I was very independent in my care, and was responsible with taking insulin and checking my blood sugar, my parents felt comfortable with me doing things on my own.

Every parent has their own parenting style. I'm not here to tell you how to parent, but I do have one recommendation: Avoid a good cop/bad cop approach. This could cause your child to sneak treats with the "good cop" and eventually whine to the "bad cop" that "Dad lets me eat a cookie after dinner when we go out to eat!" My parents were consistent in their treatment with me, so I never had the chance to do this.

Siblings

When I came home from the hospital, the entire family made changes—including my eight-year-old sister. My parents emptied the pantry, and we became an almost completely sugar-free house from that point on. There was only ever diet soda in our house. We never had Fruit Loops or Pop-Tarts around our house. It wasn't until my sister's senior year in high school that I remember there actually being Little Debbie snacks in the house. My family adjusted their diets to fit what I could eat, and this helped me feel more normal. (They still ate real desserts and such at work, at school, or whenever I wasn't around.) My father recalls thinking it was probably easier for them to shift their diet, so that I wouldn't be begging to have a bite of food I couldn't actually have.

Even though this diagnosis will affect your entire family in one way or another, don't forget about your other kids. You may find that it's easiest to clear your house of sweets, so that your child with diabetes is not tempted, or you may find that it's not necessary. If you have multiple children, consider one-on-one dinner dates, at which children who don't have diabetes can freely order dessert. Because your child with diabetes does require extra attention, be intentional about not making your other children feel left out and less important.

My sister, Tiffany, and I have talked many times about how she also became involved in taking care of me when I was younger. My parents didn't want Tiffany to feel left out, so they taught her how to help care for me. This was great because she was equipped to care for me and was always willing to go out of her way to help me.

For example, when I was in first grade, we attended the same grade school in town, but my parents both worked in neighboring towns about 30–45 minutes away. Once, my parents forgot to give me my insulin shot at breakfast, which resulted in a high blood sugar. As you know, the only way to remedy this is to take insulin, but we didn't keep any at the school since I wasn't taking insulin during the day. The school principal called my sister to the front office over the school speaker system. The school had to get special permission from my mom to let the school nurse drive Tiffany to our house to get my insulin and a syringe.

From Tiffany's perspective, these types of situations added a bit of unnecessary stress and pressure into her life. You'll need to figure out what works for your family, but I do recommend creating some boundaries so that siblings can be siblings, not just caretakers. For example, let them know that it's important to point out if they think their sibling has a low blood sugar, but it's not their job to make sure their sibling is checking their blood sugar enough.

Extended Family

Growing up, holidays were pretty normal for me. I was lucky enough to have a very loving and caring extended family. On my mother's side, both of my grandparents had diabetes. Because my mom's family was accustomed to having people with diabetes in the family, it wasn't as big of a deal to have another person with Type 1 diabetes.

My mom had eight brothers and sisters, and almost everyone would gather at my grandmother's house for the holidays each year. Everyone would bring meals, desserts, and drinks to share, and several family members made sure to bring a case of Diet Coke or bake sugar-free cookies. We did bring our own diet soda and desserts, but it meant a lot to me that my family was so inclusive.

My dad's parents were just as great. My dad only had one brother, so we were a much smaller family. I was the only person with Type 1 diabetes on this side of the family (until recent years), but that didn't matter; my grandma made sure to bake a sugar-free pie and have sugar-free ice cream on hand for me (even though others did eat it as well).

Other than desserts or diet soda, not many menu additions or adjustments need to be made, unless you know a particular food wreaks havoc on your child's blood sugars. If you have family that is not as understanding, explain to them that, for the most part, your child still eats like other children: lean meats, whole grains, and fruits and vegetables. Your family may not realize that your child feels excluded without sugar-free treats or drinks that they can have, so you can either have further conversations with them or bring your own treats. Or, your doctor may say that your child can eat a certain amount of "regular" dessert!

Even though my family was great enough to make sugar-free desserts for me around the holidays, my parents still allowed me to have a few treats. This was usually something like one cookie at dinner or a sliver of pie. Allowing these special treats is really important because it can help prevent your child from being tempted to binge eat or sneak sweets.

(Note that many recipes can be made sugar-free by replacing sugar with Splenda or stevia, or any other sugar substitute. Be cautious, though, about how many sugar-free sweets you let your child consume in one sitting. If eaten too much, sugar-free treats can sometimes cause some digestive issues, and your child may be spending their holiday in the bathroom.)

Daycare and Babysitters

Both of my parents worked full-time while I was growing up, so I had several different babysitters. None of my babysitters were professionally trained or nurses, but they all took great care of me over the years.

My mother interviewed my first babysitter in person before deciding to have her care for me. She was given lots of information about Type 1 diabetes: the testing/eating schedule that I was on, signs and symptoms of high and low blood sugars, and how to use my glucometer. I was about eight at this time, and I was already used to testing myself and was very independent. I knew what and when to eat, and knew my body well, so I could tell my babysitter if I felt like my sugars were off.

The most important thing is for your child's babysitter to have plenty of information and good communication with you as the parent. My parents always made her feel comfortable with asking questions or telling them if she was concerned about me. My mom made sure to validate her concerns and let her know she was relaying important information. (This level of communication should also apply to church group leaders, Girl Scout or Boy Scout leaders, etc.)

My second babysitter was a family friend who had a daughter my age, and my mom, again, made sure to train and equip her. The babysitter's parents also lived locally, so we would go there sometimes, and even her parents went the extra mile to have snacks that I could have on hand. It's important to talk with your child's babysitters and ask, if they are caring for your child outside of your home, if you need to provide your child's snacks or if they have appropriate snacks available.

I loved all of my babysitters! I was never skeptical of their ability to take care of me, and I was never treated as an outsider or a burden. I believe my time with my babysitters helped develop my spirit of independence, and not just because I was away from my parents. I had to learn, as a young child, to speak up for myself if I felt like my blood sugars were going too low or high—which is something I had to do many other times growing up.

Though you may not find a professionally trained childcare

provider, you could train your child's babysitter yourself, like my parents did. One of the first things you'll want to do is make sure they really understand the difference between Type 1 and Type 2 diabetes. Some people believe that Type 1 is just like Type 2 diabetes, and doesn't require much supervision beyond watching your child's diet. Some people may know a lot about Type 1 diabetes, but are still scared about their ability to manage a child's blood sugar levels while watching other children in their care.

Keep in mind that under the Americans with Disabilities Act, children who have Type 1 diabetes cannot be excluded from public and private daycare centers based on their condition. If you feel that your child is being excluded because of their diabetes, look into your state's laws and contact the American Diabetes Association's (www.diabetes.org) for info about your legal rights.

Online and In-Person Communities

Like many chronic illnesses, diabetes is an invisible monster. As much as we can try to describe how it feels to have a low or high blood sugar, it's something that has to be experienced to be fully understood. Because of this, finding a community of others who have Type 1 diabetes can be incredibly helpful.

One of the best experiences of my life was finding this community through attending a summer camp called Camp

Discovery (which you'll learn about in Chapter 7), a week-long camp only for children with Type 1 diabetes children and teenagers. If attending summer camp is not an option for your child, there are other communities available.

Facebook Groups

There is a Facebook group for just about everything. I've found groups for women with diabetes, people in my area who have diabetes, and people who use a Dexcom sensor like I do. These groups are a great place to vent frustrations or get advice from others who have experienced the same things.

Local JDRF Chapters

The Juvenile Diabetes Research Foundation (JDRF) hosts events to help raise funds to support research, education, and advocacy for individuals with Type 1 diabetes. There are a variety of events from walks and runs, bicycle races, golf competitions, and galas. Some chapters also have meetups or support groups. You can find events in your area by looking on the JDRF website. Their events are for people of all ages, not just children.

Beyond Type 1

Beyond Type 1 is a nonprofit organization that uses platforms, programs, resources, and grants to raise awareness and education about Type 1 diabetes. They have great programs to connect Type 1 diabetics, like a pen pal program, running teams, and biking teams.

Action Steps

1. Have a family meeting. What changes will take effect? What does this mean for each member in the family? If you have other children, give them a chance to ask questions.

2. Talk to your extended family about your child's diagnosis. Depending on your family situation, this could be done via email, via a phone call, or in person. You may need to talk to them again closer to holidays or family gatherings, and remind them of what your child is allowed to eat and not eat.

3. If your child will need a babysitter, begin your search, as it may take longer to find someone suitable. Care.com is a great resource to begin your search.

Chapter 5
Day-to-Day Life

...

My blood sugar went low during a family trip once, right before breakfast. We were pulling into McDonald's, so my mom said I could get a cinnamon roll. Seconds after checking, I began to re-check my blood sugar, and my mom asked what I was doing. My blood sugar was so low that I was disoriented and had already forgotten that I had just checked it.

Words can't entirely describe what low blood sugars feel like. They're scary, because you feel empty inside. You want to lie down and curl into a ball. It almost feels like an out-of-body experience. You can't think clearly or make good judgments. You get easily sidetracked, confused, angry, panicky, and shaky. You may even seem drunk to those around you. Even if your blood sugar comes back up, your body still feels off, often for another half hour. Low blood sugars can sometimes make you feel like a liability, especially at school or work.

You'll hear about many common symptoms from doctors, but everyone is different and can have their own symptoms. Over the years, I've heard of hypoglycemic symptoms, such as seeing white spots, ringing in the ears, sensitivity to light, feeling itchy, hallucinating, lips feeling tingly, or tongue going numb. I mentioned that many people with diabetes feel confused, and I've heard extreme confusion stories from other adults like not knowing where they were, not recognizing their own house or belongings, and even momentarily thinking their spouse was having an affair.

Karen Bonar, whose father has Type 1 diabetes, remembers him going low while at Disneyland with their family. After a full day of walking and family fun, and as they were on the train headed back to the hotel, her father's blood sugar dropped. Karen recalled him not being the most compliant person while low, and he started to push Karen's mom away when she tried to give him honey. Slowly and discreetly, people near them on the train inched away. When her dad still would not take anything for his low blood sugar, and became more disgruntled, people began openly avoiding "the drunk." For Karen, it was definitely embarrassing because people thought her dad (who does not drink) had become intoxicated at Disneyland!

There are many ways to treat your child's low blood sugar. Growing up, having a Capri Sun juice was my go-to remedy at home. I secretly enjoyed going low when we were out getting groceries or watching my sister's volleyball games because it usually meant I could get a regular can of soda to bring up my blood sugar. I've also treated my lows with glucose tabs, cake frosting, honey, Jolly Ranchers, and Smarties. (Once, I had a doctor who had me try slow, deep breathing during a low blood sugar to bring my levels up. It didn't work.)

While a can of regular soda was a rare "treat" for going low, the best (and worst) was going low in the middle of the night. There is a bit of an inside joke within the diabetes community about how much we eat during middle-of-the-night lows. Growing up, I always went for tortillas. I don't know why we always seemed to have them, but we did! In college, I didn't have much "extra" food around my apartment to snack on during a 2 a.m. low, so I ended up eating broccoli.

Then, there are high blood sugars. High blood sugars aren't usually such an extreme experience. Typically they cause nausea and thirstiness, but there is the risk of your child's high blood sugar leading to developing ketones or diabetic keto-acidosis (DKA). Ketones occur when the body doesn't have enough insulin. Left untreated, it can lead to DKA. I have been lucky enough to not experience this myself, but in simple terms, DKA happens when your child's body lacks insulin and begins producing extra blood acids. Your child's doctor should talk with you in-depth about how this happens, what to look for, and what to do if your child develops DKA.

As a result of long-term high blood sugars, your child may also experience a false sense of hypoglycemia. I've experienced this when my blood sugars were predominantly in the upper 100s and 200s for several months. As your child works to regulate their blood sugars, they may deal with this false sense of hypoglycemia. Their body may make them feel like they are experiencing a low blood sugar when, really, their blood sugar is only 150. It's a very frustrating experience: Your child can't drink juice to remedy a false low blood sugar, because they are not actually low. Eventually, your child's body will adjust to the new normal (where it should be), and the feeling will subside.

Occasionally, your child may also get on the blood sugar roller coaster—and it's not fun. The roller coaster begins when your child takes too much insulin for a big meal, and then their blood sugar goes low. Your child happens to over-treat their low blood sugar with too much juice or candy, and as a result, an hour later, their blood sugar goes high. So, they take insulin, and once again, their blood sugar goes low. And the cycle continues. Hopefully, they don't over-treat a second time, or take too much insulin again, but it can happen.

When your child has a low or high blood sugar, try not to jump to conclusions or accuse your child of doing something wrong. Thank your child for checking their blood sugar, and address how to correct the issue at a later time. I mentioned blood sugar logs previously, and this is another situation when having a log will be beneficial. You and your child could sit down together once a week, and look for any patterns. For example, you might point out to your child that their blood sugar rises in the late afternoon, and ask them what they are eating when they arrive home from school.

One of the most important reasons for nurturing independence in your child is because they need to own this diagnosis. Diabetes does not own them. Nor does it define them. This is hard to teach your child, because Type 1 diabetes is a 24-hours-a-day, all-consuming condition.

Different Factors that Affect Blood Sugars

High blood sugars, low blood sugars, and everything in between—what can cause your child's blood sugars to fluctuate? Obviously, food and insulin are the biggest factors. But many other things can impact blood sugar levels. Some of the these may not ever affect your child, or may do so only temporarily, but they are things to be aware of, just in case. Keep in mind this is not an exhaustive list.

Diabetes does not own them. Nor does it define them.

Specific Foods
You may find that anytime your child eats a particular food or meal, their blood sugar skyrockets. High-carb foods like pizza and pasta do seem to affect a lot of people with Type 1 diabetes, but there's a chance those foods won't affect your

child. Other foods that have been known to cause issues for some individuals include oatmeal, applesauce, and even drinks with caffeine. It's totally a case-by-case basis, so you'll just need to watch for patterns.

Holidays

During special occasions like holidays or family reunions, people tend to eat more—including your child. It's also pretty likely that your family doesn't eat your "typical" (everyday) foods for holidays and other special occasions. With different foods and bigger portions, the holidays can cause some problems with your child's blood sugars. Talk to your child's doctor about how to prepare for the holidays, as they may have you increase their long-acting insulin or increase their basal rates on their insulin pump.

Emotions

The first week of school can be exciting and stressful for any child, and children with Type 1 diabetes can especially struggle during this time. Any stressful, emotional, or high-pressure situation can cause some blood sugar issues. Whether it's a breakup, taking a big test, losing a puppy, fighting with friends, or moving schools, be prepared for fluctuating blood sugars.

Puberty

As if puberty isn't enough to deal with by itself, it's also makes diabetes management more difficult. The physical growth that happens during puberty is usually accompanied by an increased need for insulin. Like most kids, your child will likely want to eat more food. It's important to stay aware of what they eat so they take the right amount of insulin to cover the food. During this time, you'll also want to consult with your child's doctor more often.

Being Sick
Whether it's a head cold or the flu, being sick is another factor that can affect your child's blood sugars. It's extra stress on the body, not to mention that your child is probably not eating as much and might be dehydrated. Some medicines (both over-the-counter and prescription) can also raise your child's blood sugars. Be sure to talk with your child's doctor before giving them any medicine, and discuss how to handle your child's sick days.

Fitting In

As someone with Type 1 diabetes, your child may not always feel like they fit in with their classmates or friends. They may not feel normal like their peers. Children with Type 1 diabetes can feel especially left out during holiday and birthday parties. Some parents are more lenient and let their children have sweets occasionally, while other parents don't. My parents were the latter, which meant I got crunchy granola bars or Fruit Roll-Ups at parties.

Sometimes this desire to be normal can result in dangerous decisions like lying about their blood sugars, just to be allowed to eat a special treat. It's important that you verify your child's blood sugars, especially in instances when they want a treat. As a fourth grader, I lied to my mom about my blood sugar so that she would let me eat a few pieces of candy at our Valentine's Day party. A little white lie like this could land your child in the hospital.

There were many parties where I was given the granola bars, instead of a sweet treat, and just wouldn't eat them. Cupcakes and granola bars are not comparable! Some classroom parents were very accommodating and brought me my own sugar-free treat, and sometimes my parents made me a sugar-free treat. To help your child feel less awkward, it's also helpful if your child's treat is served at the same time as everyone else's.

If your child is going to be at a school party, why not find a recipe online and bake some sugar-free treats instead of sending granola bars? Kids already miss out on desserts at lunch, and letting them have a semi-sweet treat at a party is one less time they might feel "different" at school. If you can pack your child's lunch and include a dessert, that would be better and probably healthier, and this can help establish healthy food relationships.

Weight Loss

Trying to lose weight as someone with Type 1 diabetes—whether as a teenager or an adult—can be incredibly difficult. This, in part, is because insulin prevents the breakdown of fat cells and stimulates the creation of body fat. This does not mean that insulin is literally making your child fatter every time they take their insulin; insulin just makes weight loss a little complicated.

If you research how people with Type 1 diabetes can try to lose weight, you'll probably come across a low-carb, high-fat diet (LCHF). Similarly, there is also a ketogenic diet, which has stricter guidelines than just eating foods that are low-carb. Individuals with Type 1 diabetes take insulin when they eat carbs, but there are foods that are extremely low-carbo-hydrate—meats and vegetables, mainly. (Some people with Type 1 diabetes may also require insulin when eating protein or fat. Your child's doctor will discuss this with you.) If your child eats fewer carbs throughout their day, they won't need to take as much insulin.

Both of these diets should be approached with extreme caution. If your child is physically active, this diet could be causing more harm than good, because it might lead to an inadequate fuel supply; carbohydrates need to be present for most people. Please remember it's important to consult your child's physician before changing their diet or eating habits. This is especially important when your child is still young, because a ketogenic diet can affect their growth.

Following a low-carb diet is not the only option for losing weight. As your child gets older, working with a personal trainer and/or registered dietitian to help them lose weight could be something to consider. I have worked with a personal trainer for a few years to help me get in better shape and lose weight. I was not put on any type of restrictive diet and have still been able to lose weight.

If you are looking to modify any recipes, consider using substitutes like almond or coconut flour. There are also many baking recipes that use ingredients like avocados or sugar-free applesauce. Though your child may not actually need to follow a specific meal plan, looking into ketogenic, vegan, or paleo recipes could be helpful in maintaining better blood sugar control.

There is another way that your child may try to lose weight, and it also involves taking less insulin. Intentionally taking a lot less insulin than needed to try to lose weight is called diabulimia, and it is extremely dangerous. As I previously mentioned, insulin promotes fat storage. Without insulin, the body can't break down food into sugar, and has to feed off fat, muscles, and organs for energy.

Diabulimia can have severe consequences, such as diabetic

ketoacidosis, retinopathy, neuropathy, stroke, and even death. Talk to your child's doctor about what to look for and how to prevent your child from developing diabulimia. Your child's doctor may also recommend consulting with a psychologist or behaviorist.

Diabetes and Sports

Being physically active can help with weight loss, and improved overall health, but exercise can cause low blood sugars. This can make playing sports with Type 1 diabetes a little challenging—not impossible, just challenging. I always played volleyball, which starts at the beginning of the school year. The first week of practice was kind of a "shock" to my body. Even though I spent summers semi-active between swimming and riding my bike, that was nothing compared to running laps during volleyball practice.

Before your child begin playing any sports, it's important to talk to your child's coaches and endocrinologist. It would be beneficial to first talk to the coach, and get an idea of how long practices will last and what they might entail. With this information in hand, you can form a game plan with how to adjust snacks and insulin levels before and after practices and games.

There were many practices when I had to sit on the sidelines because of a low or high blood sugar. This was tough for me, because not only did I not feel great physically, but emotionally I wanted to be out there with my teammates.

My teammates never said anything to me directly, nor do I think they voiced anything to my coaches, but I overheard comments about me faking a low blood sugar (to get out of practice) in the hallway and locker room. I didn't say anything, mostly because I felt my coaches were also frustrated by me having to sit out. This is why it's important to include coaches in your yearly 504 plan meetings (more on this in Chapter 6), and really stress the effects that exercise has on blood sugars.

When teams had to travel to other schools for games, athletes were provided a light meal, usually a sandwich, chips, and a granola bar. (I could not escape those granola bars!) Eating beforehand can help sustain your child through the games, so their blood sugar is less likely to drop. It is a tricky situation when you mix food, exercise, and insulin. Exercise lowers blood sugars, but food raises blood sugars. There may be a lot of trial and error, so open communication with your child's doctor will be important.

We also had a few volleyball tournaments every year, which meant playing five or six games on a Saturday. These tournament days were fun, but also challenging. Team moms would often make snacks and cookies for everyone to help refuel our energy between games. Just like everyone else, I needed to refuel, but I had to be smart about my snack choices. I still needed to take insulin to cover this food, but I didn't want to take too much and go low.

If your child is interested in sports, don't hold them back due to your own fear. Many professional athletes are active with Type 1 diabetes: Jay Cutler is a NFL quarterback, Gary Hall, Jr. was an Olympic gold-medal swimmer, and Kelli Kuehne was an American pro golfer. It's safe to say that these athletes endure more physical activity than a high school sports practice.

Allison Caggia, the Editorial Director at Diabetes Daily, has Type 1 diabetes and enjoys CrossFit workouts, which can be more strenuous than typical gym workout routines. To keep her blood sugars in check, she eats a low-carb meal before her CrossFit workout each day. Allison realized that high-intensity interval workouts and weightlifting would cause her blood sugars to spike after the workout, so she now takes one unit of insulin just minutes before she begins a workout, so that the insulin starts to kick in toward the end of her workout and bring her blood sugar back into the normal range.

It took both Allison and me some trial and error to figure out what works for us before, during, and after exercise. The most important thing is to always have insulin on hand in case of high blood sugars, and glucose tabs or some kind of sugar on hand to treat low blood sugars. If you are nervous about your child's blood sugars and exercise, start with something low-key like riding a bike around the neighborhood with them.

Burnout

Diabetes burnout is a very real thing. Your child may not experience it until adulthood, but it's not out of the question for a child to feel burnout, and it's something you'll want to talk about with them at some point so they know how to handle it when it happens. William Polonsky's book *Diabetes Burnout: What to Do When You Can't Take it Anymore* is a great in-depth resource on this subject.

Keeping Type 1 diabetes in consistent, good control takes a lot of intentional effort—and it can be exhausting. After many, many years, sometimes people with Type 1 diabetes lose the motivation to keep everything in control. During a period of burnout, people with Type 1 diabetes can begin to ignore certain parts of their care (checking blood sugars less often, not taking insulin, etc.).

Burnout is important to address, because it could potentially also lead to depression. According to the American Diabetes Association, there is no definitive link between diabetes and depression, but people with Type 1 diabetes are at a higher risk for developing depression. As someone who has suffered with depression unrelated to my diabetes, I can attest to the fact that depression, regardless of the reason, can affect your child's diabetes management.

Experiencing burnout and depression can also lead to

Keeping Type 1 diabetes in consistent, good control takes a lot of intentional effort—and it can be exhausting.

people with Type 1 diabetes not feeling up for the fight. While I've never personally experienced this high level of burnout, I have heard others who have. It's difficult for them to even want to get out of bed. You may think this just sounds like depression, but it reaches another level of danger when someone with Type 1 diabetes doesn't want to get out of bed to treat a low blood sugar.

One way to help your child during a period of burnout is to limit the number of decisions they have to make in a day. This practice also lends itself to helping you avoid something called decision fatigue. Coined by psychologist Roy F. Baumeister, decision fatigue is something many people experience after they make decision after decision all day, and eventually become so tired of making decisions that they start making poor decisions or feel they can't make a decision at all. For example, have you ever come home from work, and had no idea what you want for dinner, and can't make a decision because your brain just feels . . . empty? It's likely you're experiencing decision fatigue.

As individuals with Type 1 diabetes, we have even more decisions to make throughout each day than others do. Do I want to count this lunch as 30 carbs or 40 carbs? Should I eat cheese or crackers before my workout? Should I change my pump site before or after dinner? One way that my husband and I cut down on daily decisions is meal prepping. Every Saturday, we fix our meals for the week, and eat the same breakfast, lunch, dinner, and snacks for one week. So, I might decide that for one week, I will eat a burrito bowl for lunch every day. I'll figure out the serving sizes of each ingredient and add up the carbs so I know how much insulin to take at lunch. Then, for the rest of the week, I don't really have to put much thought to my lunch bolus, since I know it will be the same every day.

If your child is still living at home and you believe they are experiencing burnout, consider putting them on a "diabetic vacation" for a few days. This is not a true vacation; it just means that you take over all control of diabetes care. This break should be not only a relief, but also show them that even when their parents are in control, blood sugars can still go haywire. When they see this happening, it may help relieve them of guilt or pressure about their diabetes care.

Another thing that can help prevent burnout from occurring is talking with your child about expectations and letting them know they don't have to be perfect. In can also be beneficial to have "off" days built into your year. Since I was diagnosed so young, my doctors advised my parents to give me three or four days a year to just be a kid.

Halloween, Thanksgiving, Christmas, and my birthday were our chosen "off" days. These "off" days were not a total free-for-all. For instance, on Halloween night, I was allowed to eat a few pieces of candy. Unbeknownst to me, my parents would eat some of my candy, and then throw some away. I would get to eat a little more candy the next day, and again, my parents would eat some, and throw some away. This way, I was still able to eat candy (as were my parents!), but not an excessive amount. I was able to be a normal kid with my friends, even if for just one night.

Another pseudo-holiday that I started celebrating in college was my "diabetic birthday" (sometimes called a *dia-versary*). Growing up, each year on July 4th, my parents would say something about it being my diabetic birthday, but there was no celebration. Thanks to social media, I noticed that my friends who also had diabetes were celebrating their diabetic birthday (something like going out for dinner or getting ice cream). Now, every year I do the same. I choose to celebrate this day because it marks another year of hard work and, honestly, survival. This is a simple tradition you could start early on with your child!

Whether they experience burnout at a young age or once they're on their own, seeing a licensed counselor can be really beneficial. As I've pointed out throughout the book, many facets go into dealing with diabetes on a daily basis. Talking to an unbiased person can be good to work through the burnout and learn more healthy coping mechanisms.

Action Steps

1. Make a mental note to track any fluctuations in your child's blood sugars and what may have caused the change.

2. Start trying some different recipes for treats so that your child has a few favorites to pick from for school parties and other occasions when one might be needed.

3. In your calendar or planner, write down your child's date of diagnosis, so you can celebrate their "diabetic birthday" next year. If you use Google Calendar, you can make the event automatically repeat each year, so you never forget.

Chapter 6
School and Diabetes

...

The summer before I started third grade, my family moved to a new town. During the first week of school, the school nurse read *Taking Diabetes to School* by Kim Gosselin to my entire class. She talked to them about what to expect and what to do, explained that diabetes is not like cooties, and answered questions.

Let's be honest: I don't know how well my third-grade classmates comprehended this information. Later that year, one classmate didn't want to sit next to me on the bus because she didn't want to "catch diabetes from me."

Thankfully, by the time high school started, my classmates weren't bothered by my diabetes. In fact, they almost had an interest in it at times. For safety, I always took a buddy with me to the nurse's office when I had a low blood sugar; no one wanted me to faint in the hallway alone. I was not "popular" among the boys in my class, but they were usually most eager to go with me—because it meant getting out of class for five minutes.

504 Plans

At the beginning of each school year, my mom scheduled a meeting with the head cafeteria cook, the principal, the school nurse, and my classroom teachers. Typically, both parents or guardians are involved, but my mom worked at the school, so it was easier for her to take the lead. We lived in a very small town, so my mom was able to get the meetings set up by herself. (If your school is being uncooperative, there is a small chance you may need the assistance of a lawyer or to call American Diabetes Association to intercede.) During this meeting, my mom had information on hand to give to everyone: what I could and could not have, what to do when I was low, what to do when I was high, handling emergency situations, and more. This meeting was required by my 504 plan.

What is a 504 plan? According to Understood.org, it's a legally binding document that helps prevent discrimination, and provide necessary accommodations in public school districts, institutions of higher education, and other state and local education agencies, for individuals with disabilities. To get your child a 504 plan at their school, contact the school principal or guidance counselor to get the process started. They will need a written request formally asking for a 504 plan for your child. The school may also request paperwork that shows an official diagnosis of your child's Type 1 diabetes.

The school administrators will then have a meeting to discuss if a 504 plan is suitable for your child, and what accommodations they think are necessary to include. Because you are the best advocate for your child, it's important that you be a part of this meeting. You know your child better than anyone else, and you need to be there to voice your concerns and opinions. You'll want to be sure to cover all of your bases: classes, tests, snacks, and even field trips.

Each 504 plan is different, depending on what you ask for and what the school is willing to do. (You can even make specific requests, like not serving your child a hardboiled egg as a snack every day. Extra thanks for that, Mom!) Some mandates that I would strongly consider including in your child's 504 plan are that the school provide daily snacks and a lunch calendar ahead of time. If your child is still in grade school, it may also be beneficial to have a paraprofessional at the school come into class and check your child's blood sugar. Younger children can be more forgetful or may feel too embarrassed to do it themselves in the middle of class. In grade school, I had a paraprofessional who checked my blood sugar (at the back of the classroom) and gave me a snack. Once I reached junior high, I took full responsibility to check my blood sugar and get my snacks.

504 plans are also there to save the day when your child's blood sugars interfere with their learning. In third grade I failed a spelling test, and I had not struggled with spelling before. My teacher later brought up the test score at a parent-teacher conference, and it surprised my mom. She went home, looked back at my blood sugars, and found that I had gone low about the same time as the test. Thanks to my 504 plan, I was able to retake the test. From then on, we knew to pay closer attention to blood sugars before tests and even when doing homework.

Even with a 504 plan in place, there will likely be a few hiccups along the way. My mom wrote out a monthly menu for the cooks to follow as they prepared my lunch, with specific portions written out and desserts usually left off of my tray. Once, when I was in fourth grade, I was accidentally served a kolache dessert roll. Instead of asking if it was correct for me to get one, I assumed my mom was finally going to let me eat a dessert! I kept my mouth shut, found a seat at a table, and ate that kolache before anything else on my tray.

Of course, the cooks realized their mistake and told the teacher who was on cafeteria duty to go get the dessert from my tray. Imagine their surprise when it had already been eaten. I was given a stern lecture about knowing better than to eat the dessert. (Can you blame me, though?) There is no leniency or "just this once" with a 504 plan in place!

There may also be situations when you realize the 504 plan is lacking instructions. For example, when I was in fifth grade, I had to start taking insulin shots before lunch. The school allowed me to choose one friend to go with me each day, so I didn't have to stand in the lunch line alone—that is, until someone complained because they weren't being chosen. My options were to let every student in the class have a turn or to go alone. Because this is was a new development in my care, it wasn't outlined in the 504 plan. You should have a yearly meeting to discuss your child's 504 plan so that you can make adjustments as needed. If more serious updates are needed sooner, you may ask for additional meetings.

504 plans are still applicable at certain colleges and universities. Your child will need to set this plan up with the college themselves, and their plan from high school may not transfer. I actually did not know this information when I went to college, nor did I feel that I needed to have the plan in place. But, if your child would like a plan in place, they'll need to contact the disability office on campus, prove their condition, and fill out paperwork, and then they'll have official information to provide to their professors. This paperwork will outline necessary information and accommodations, such as that your child may need to reschedule exams in the event of a low blood sugar.

504 Plans vs. IEPs

According to Understood.org, an individualized education

program (IEP) provides special education services because the child has a disability that affects their performance and/or ability to learn like others. Meanwhile, a 504 plan provides services and changes to the learning environment, because their disability may interfere with their learning.

Because your child's Type 1 diabetes may only occasionally interfere with their classroom experience, the plan acts as "if this, then that" support. For example, the plan might state that your child is allowed to participate in physical education class and sports, but teachers and coaches must make sure necessary supplies and treatment are on -hand, and be fully trained to treat low blood sugars.

Action Steps

1. If your child is in school, call the school to start the process of setting up a 504 plan. Start thinking about what accommodations you want in place for your child.

2. If you will be training any school employees, begin preparing what you will talk about. If the school nurse will be doing the training, verify that he or she has the right information regarding your child's snacks, insulin dosages, etc.

Chapter 7
Camp, Traveling, and Being Away from Home

...

Like many chronic illnesses, diabetes is an invisible monster. As much as we can try to describe how it feels to have a low or high blood sugar, it's something that has to be experienced to be fully understood. Because of this, finding a community of others with Type 1 diabetes can be incredibly helpful.

One of the best experiences of my life was finding this community through attending a summer camp called Camp Discovery, a week-long camp only for children with Type 1 diabetes children and teenagers. I attended as a camper for more than 15 years and then became a camp counselor. A lot of kids come to Camp Discovery from small rural communities where they're the only one with Type 1 diabetes, so part of camp is being able to shake off that "freak" status.

Every week at camp included the typical summer camp mix

of indoor and outdoor activities. Younger campers in the first week had a schedule to follow, whereas older campers in the second week could choose their activities each day.

The main indoor activity was the education sessions, at which the doctors and nurses taught us different things like how to refine our carb-counting skills, how to deal with mean kids at school, and even how to give ourselves our own insulin shots. At the older kids' camp, there was also a Q&A time with counselors to get more insight about dealing with diabetes and college, jobs, etc.

All in all, it was just a typical week of summer camp, where children with Type 1 diabetes could be around others just like themselves, eat peanuts and raisins, and help each other count carbs. Camp wouldn't be camp without some special events like the big scavenger hunt, Olympic races, talking to "Aunt FiFi" (a counselor with a megaphone on the other side of the building), and the Kiss-a-Pig competition.

Kiss-a-Pig Competition

The purpose of the Kiss-a-Pig competition was to increase awareness about diabetes and the American Diabetes Association, and to raise funds to support the American Diabetes Association. A pig was used because it was one of the first sources of insulin.

Each year, before camp, campers were given a fundraising sheet to collect donations for the Kiss-a-Pig competition. People made donations to the American Diabetes Association, and campers received points (that turned into stickers) based on the amount raised. Each camp counselor had a poster with their name on it hanging in the cafeteria at camp. Campers would place their stickers on the posters of who they wanted to kiss a pig. If a camper raised $100, they got 100 stickers, and they could place them on whichever counselor (or counselors) poster they wanted.

At the end of the week, the counselors with the most stickers had to literally kiss a pig. There were a few years when a pig could not be found, so one of the camp doctors would dress up in a pig costume! During one of my last years as a counselor, instead of a pig, we had to kiss a dog. (This sounds less scary for most people, but I was terrified of dogs at the time.)

The American Diabetes Association and Juvenile Diabetes Research Foundation both host events to help raise funds to support research, education, and advocacy for individuals with Type 1 diabetes. There are a variety of events from walks and runs, bicycle races, golf competitions, and galas. You can find events in your area by looking on the American Diabetes Association and Juvenile Diabetes Research Foundation websites.

What I Gained from Going to Camp

The biggest lesson I learned during all of my years at camp was that I was in control—that diabetes did not control me. To stay healthy and alive, I had to become more independent with my diabetes care, own it, and show it who was boss. I also believe that spending a week away from my parents, and being taught how to better care for myself, helped me become the strong, independent woman I am today.

As we got older, we were also more in charge of our insulin intake. Every camper would take insulin before they got in line to eat, and a nurse would help them withdraw the right amount. Nurses and doctors would ask older campers if we felt like we needed to adjust our insulin based on that evening's planned events. The camp staff wasn't there to spoil us; they were there to help teach us and help us better manage our Type 1 diabetes.

Bob Hamrick, a longtime Camp Discovery counselor, recalled a story from a camper's mother. A mother was picking up her son from Camp Discovery, and told Bob that the first time her son had spent a night away from home was as a second-grader at the camp. Keeping him safe, she thought, meant keeping him in sight. Finally, she agreed to give Camp Discovery a try. She told Bob, "When we turned the hill, you could see all these kids. My son had the door opened before I could even stop, and he turned to me and said, 'Look, Mom!

Kids just like me!' and ran off. I sat and cried, and felt pretty stupid until I looked around at all the other cars, with parents sitting there, wiping their own tears. And I thought, '**Look— mommies and daddies, just like me.**'"

The best part of attending this camp for 15 years was that I got to spend time around other children with Type 1 diabetes and just feel "normal" for a few days. I didn't have to quietly get someone's attention to tell them that I felt low. I didn't have to be the weird one eating sugar-free ice cream while others got "real" desserts. I built lifelong friends at these camps, like Ellie, who was a bridesmaid in my wedding.

Camp wasn't the only time that I was away from my parents for more than a few hours. On the way home from a yearbook workshop in high school, we stopped at Sonic to get lunch. We got our food and continued home because I had a softball game to play in that evening. Little did I know, the Diet Dr Pepper I ordered turned out to not be diet after all. Drinking 32 ounces of regular Dr Pepper wreaks havoc on blood sugars. Luckily, I didn't go into diabetic ketoacidosis (DKA), as that would have meant a hospital visit. I did feel nauseous, though, and I scared my yearbook advisor half to death.

Receiving the wrong drink order has happened numerous times. Sometimes I'm able to tell right away and just can walk up to the counter to get a new drink. It's important that your child have the confidence to speak up for themselves—which is not always easy to do when they're with a group of friends.

Getting the wrong drink happened just recently at a fast-food restaurant, and they had confirmed the drink order before handing it to my husband and me. It tasted off, so when I got home, I used my glucometer to test the drink. Instead of sticking a drop of blood on the strip, I used a drop of soda. The glucometer read "HI," which meant my soda was not diet. I called the restaurant and kindly let them know what happened. To most people, a wrong drink order is just annoying, but it can have severe consequences for someone with Type 1 diabetes.

Simple situations like this happening close to home can make traveling with Type 1 diabetes seem scary, but it's not impossible. I've done international vacations, mission trips with lots of activity, amusement parks, and everything in between. Like everything else, you and your child will be used to it after a few trips!

Planes, Trains, and Automobiles

During college, I started to travel more. The first few times were a bit nerve-wracking for me, because I was traveling without my parents. I wondered what would happen if my blood sugars went awry, or how I would handle things being even further away from my parents. Thankfully, my family had traveled when I was younger, so it wasn't entirely unfamiliar to me—and I never had any issues. I love to travel, and still do it often.

Another detail that can make traveling complicated is a time change. Depending on how big the time change is, you might see a small spike in your child's blood sugars. Time changes can cause problems, for example, if your child's blood sugars are lower in the afternoon and their insulin pump settings are set accordingly. When your child's pump thinks it's the afternoon, but it's actually late in the evening, it could cause a high blood sugar due to the lower insulin levels. If a trip will be longer than two days, I usually keep my insulin pump clock the same for the first day, and then adjust the time to match the time of where we're visiting. This is definitely a situation that you will want to talk to your child's doctor about before leaving for your trip.

Road trips are a little easier because you probably don't have to deal with time change, and you definitely don't deal with any airport security issues. As someone who flies a few times a year, I'll warn you that most airport security agents believe an insulin pump and continuous glucose monitor (CGM) can go through a body scanner, while most insulin pump manufacturing companies say they can't.

Specifically, here are the airport guidelines for a few different devices:

- Medtronic's website states, "You can continue to wear your insulin pump or continuous glucose monitor (CGM) while going through common security systems such as an airport metal detector as it will not harm the device or trigger an alarm. Do not send the devices through the x-ray machine. You need to remove your insulin pump and CGM (sensor and transmitter) while going through an airport body scanner."

- Omnipod's website states, "Pod and PDMs can safely pass through airport X-ray machines. The Pod and PDM can tolerate common electromagnetic and electrostatic fields, including airport security and cellular phones."

- Tandem's website states, "Tandem insulin pump should NOT be put through machines that use X-rays, including airline luggage X-ray machines and full-body scanners."

- Dexcom's website states, "When wearing your G6, ask for hand-wanding or a full-body pat down and visual inspection instead of going through the Advanced Imaging Technology (AIT) body scanners (also called a millimeter wave scanner). Don't put your Dexcom G6 CGM System components through x-ray machines."

- Freestyle Libre's website states, "Some airport full-body scanners include x-ray or millimeter radio-wave, which you cannot expose your System to. The effect of these scanners has not been evaluated and the exposure may damage the System or cause inaccurate results."

So, it's safe to say that it's recommended to only go through a metal detector with a pump or CGM, or get a pat-down from the TSA. I find it easiest to always allow for a little extra time and request a pat-down during each visit to the airport.

If your child does not have a pump or CGM, TSA regulations state that you will need to carry their syringes and insulin vials together with a pharmacy label that clearly identifies the medication. Never store insulin in checked luggage, because it may be exposed to extreme (often freezing) temperatures, which can change its effectiveness. It's also better to have it in your carry-on so, if the airline loses your luggage, you still have your child's insulin. You'll also want to carry a glucagon in its pharmacy-labeled container. If you are bringing extra lancets, they will need to be capped and carried along with your child's glucometer. Should you have any difficulties when trying to pass through airport security, Medtronic's website recommends you ask to speak with the TSA ground security commissioner.

I've traveled internationally without problems, but not everyone is as lucky. Heather Wilkins, another individual with Type 1 diabetes, had to take a trip to the emergency room while visiting London, because she got the flu. Luckily, she was able to receive some medicine to help her recover for her trip back to the States. During that visit she learned that people with Type 1 diabetes in America use different units when measuring blood sugar levels than those living in Europe. According to the American Diabetes Association, most blood sugar test results are reported as mmol/L (millimoles per liter–) outside of the United States. In the United States, blood sugars are shown as mg/dL (milligrams per deciliter).

Ellie Hook, who I've mentioned previously, has traveled abroad several times and also hasn't always had the best luck. In fact, once her insulin pump stopped working right before she ventured into the Amazon rainforest. Because there are so many barriers to getting a new pump while abroad (phoning an international number, time differences, short stays at one address, language barriers, etc.), she tried to get long-acting insulin at a local pharmacy to supplement her short-acting insulin and used manual shots for the duration of the trip. Simultaneously, she had the manufacturing company ship a replacement pump to her home address so it would be waiting for her when she returned. (Most insulin pump companies will actually provide a backup pump for international travel to take with you. You just call to make the arrangements ahead of time.)

Packing for Your Trip

When I was younger, I took three bags on every trip: my suitcase, my glucometer and insulin purse, and a soft cooler bag for snacks. There are several things to consider while you're packing and planning.

Snacks

Your child will need some snacks to have on hand during your trip. You'll want a variety of snacks, but don't forget to have some kind of protein snack. Cheese sticks and beef jerky are great options because they aren't messy. Peanut butter is a good option to have available for when you are back at the hotel.

Cooler

Insulin, glucometers, and test strips need to stay at room temperature. If you're also storing drinks and have ice packs in the cooler, do not allow any of the medical supplies to touch the ice packs. If you get out of the car at a rest stop or restaurant, be sure to take all the medical supplies inside with you so that they don't get too hot or cold.

Sugar

Inevitably, your child's blood sugar will go low, so you need to have some kind of sugar on hand. Juice boxes are great for the car or a hotel room. If you'll be out and about, juice boxes aren't as handy, so try to have glucose tablets or hard candy. Depending on where you'll be, you might be able to run into a convenience store or restaurant and grab a regular soda, too.

Diabetes Supplies

You will, of course, need a glucometer, test strips, insulin bottles (or pens), and needles. If your child is on an insulin pump, you'll also want to take extra insulin needles, in case the pump stops working during your trip. The Transportation Security Administration (TSA) advises individuals with diabetes to carry insulin in the original, labeled box from the pharmacy. You'll also want to be sure and include their glucagon.

Always be sure to take extra pump supplies, because you never know when bad weather might strike and keep you from getting home on time. Most home pharmacies can (and will) send a prescription to wherever you and your child are, but that won't help when it comes to insulin pump supplies. If you are going overseas, and your child wears an insulin pump, I recommend also getting a long-acting insulin (like Lantus) to also have on hand.

Doctor's Note

If you are traveling overseas, carry a doctor's note that says your child is a Type 1 diabetic and needs the medical supplies that you are carrying with you. Airport security agents may not even ask for it or look for it, but better safe than sorry. A letter isn't necessary when traveling domestically but is still recommended as a precaution.

Diabetes and Driving

While we're on the topic of travel, it's important to also talk about what to do when your child is ready to start driving.

Individuals with Type 1 diabetes safely drive their cars every day, and your child can do the same.

It's always a smart idea for your child to check their blood sugar before getting behind the wheel. It's never safe for your child to drive while their blood sugar is out of range, especially if it is low. This is especially true because if your child is low and pulled over by a police officer, there is a chance they could be accused of driving under the influence, since the symptoms of low blood sugar and being intoxicated are very similar.

When your child begins driving, they should always keep something in the car to treat low blood sugars: glucose tabs, Gatorade, granola bars, peanuts, etc. My purse is always full of hard candies, the middle console in my car contains snacks, and I have additional snacks in my trunk. I also keep spare change in my car in case I run out of treatment options in my car and need to buy something. (I do have a debit card, but I keep change on hand in case my only option is a vending machine.)

Every state has different licensing laws and policies for people with Type 1 diabetes. You and your child can easily look up this information on the American Diabetes Association website.

Action Steps

1. Consider looking into a summer camp for children with Type 1 diabetes. Enrollment usually starts several months in advance!

2. Buy a bag (or two) for your child to carry their supplies with them when needed. Visit www.thetype1life.com for resources.

Chapter 8
Diabetes as an Adult

...

I wondered why I couldn't move.

After a few minutes, I somehow forced my arm to nudge my husband, Aaron, enough to wake him. "I can't move," I told him. He was half-asleep and didn't understand what I meant, so I repeated myself and also noted that I thought my blood sugar was low.

He hurried to the kitchen to get honey and then tried to hand it to me when he walked back in our bedroom. With tears streaming down my face, I told him he needed to put the honey in my mouth. I had lived 21 years with Type 1 diabetes, but I had never experienced this feeling before.

We waited for the honey to kick in and to see if I would start to feel normal again. Instead, it got worse. I tried to talk, but my speech was intermittent and slurred. I knew what I wanted to say, but the words wouldn't form. Terrified, I stared at Aaron with tears in my eyes, trying to will my mouth to move. He was equally terrified, as his wild-eyed wife just silently, and intently, stared at him, at 2 o'clock in the morning of my 25th birthday. He was truly scared, as I had never had a low blood sugar make me act that way.

Eventually, I communicated to Aaron to call my sister. I'm not sure why I wanted him to do this, as I still couldn't form words much. She urged Aaron to not wait it out, but instead to take me to the emergency room.

By the time we arrived at the ER, I was a bit more coherent. But then, things got worse again. I was acting so erratic that the doctors asked Aaron if I had taken drugs, and ordered blood work to verify that I had not. I was admitted and spent a few days in the hospital, and lots of tests were run. While the main reason I ended up there was a low blood sugar, how everything happened concerned the doctors.

The doctors never reached a conclusion, but they did think part of what contributed to this scary event was stress. Five months prior, I unexpectedly lost my mom in a car wreck, so I was dealing with a lot of grief and depression. This was my first birthday without my mom, and in a few weeks, I was to bury my mom's ashes. Stress has always had an effect on my blood sugars, and the doctors believed it just built up to be too much for my system.

After being discharged, I visited more doctors, in part because for several weeks after I was discharged, I couldn't eat anything and kept getting sick. I saw both a neurologist and gastroenterologist, with still no solution. For a few weeks, they thought I had gastroesophageal reflux disease (GERD), but that turned out to not be the case. To this day, we don't know for sure what happened or how I got better.

Looking back, going to these different doctors was the perfect example of me being my own advocate. If it weren't for my parents teaching me to advocate for my own health, I may not have gone through all of that to try to find answers. I wasn't so sure that it was just a stress-related issue, and I only stopped going to the different doctors for testing when all the symptoms subsided. (Coincidentally, I began to feel better the day after we got our first dog. Perhaps, in the end, it was a stress-related issue that needed some puppy love?)

College Life

My father said that sending me to college was very hard, because he and my mom didn't want me to go too far in case something happened. But by the time I went to college, I already had 15 years of experience handling my diabetes, mostly on my own. Thankfully, my parents trusted me and were confident that I understood the gravity of my situation.

When I went to college, I didn't tell every single person that I had Type 1 diabetes. I told the resident assistant in my dorm, my roommate, and a few of my professors. Just like in grade school, more and more people found out over time. I told them when it was appropriate or if I felt they needed to know.

Most of my college friends just knew I had Type 1 diabetes and that was it. Some of my close friends took extra concern, and actually learned more about Type 1 diabetes and what to do in emergency situations. Again, not everyone I was around needed to know what to do. My best friends were the people I was around the most, and therefore the ones who knew the most about my diabetes.

As I mentioned previously, 504 plans are still applicable in certain colleges. Your child will need to set this plan up with the college themselves, and their plan from high school may not transfer.

You'll also want to remind your child to list you as a contact on their HIPAA release forms. This is important, so that you can access medical information and forms if needed. Not being a legal professional, I'm not going to dive in too deep about legal topics. The American Diabetes Association has lots of information available about laws to protect your child, HIPAA, power of attorney, and much more.

Alcohol

According to the American Diabetes Association, alcohol can cause a drop in blood sugar levels. The 2015 Youth Risk Behavior Survey found that 33% of high school students drank some amount of alcohol in the last 30 days—and your child may be one of those students someday. Even if not, they'll turn 21 eventually and will need to know how to handle alcohol if they choose to drink.

Because of the impact that alcohol has on blood sugars, it's important for your child to eat something along with their alcohol and check their blood sugar more often than usual after drinking. It can get a little more complicated if they get a drink like a margarita or daiquiri that has lots of sugar in it, as the alcohol lowers blood sugar levels but the sugar raises levels. It's taken some trial and error for me to figure out the best solution for me, and your child will want to consult their doctor for specific advice.

Doctors recommend that your child wear some type of diabetes identification in general, but especially when they may be drinking alcohol. The symptoms of too much alcohol and a low blood sugar can be similar, and you don't want friends (or strangers) brushing off your child as just being too intoxicated. For this reason, I've always made sure that I'm not alone during or after drinking. (You can find medical ID resources at www.thetype1life.com.)

Marriage

Diabetes is a life-altering disease. Your child can live a happy, fulfilling life with it, no doubt. But it is something that requires a lot of attention to detail. When I was younger, I remember wondering if there would be a man who would even want to have a wife with Type 1 diabetes.

I don't remember the specific details of how I told my husband, Aaron, that I have Type 1 diabetes. I do remember having some conversations with him, during which he asked lots of questions about my diabetes. It never seemed to phase him in the slightest. From Aaron's perspective, marrying someone with diabetes was never intimidating or scary. We dated for two years, so we had plenty of conversations about the ups and downs of diabetes. Because I was honest and transparent about my diabetes, his expectations and the reality of living with someone with Type 1 diabetes were the same.

One important conversation that your child will need to have with their significant other is the element of accountability. Aaron cares for me deeply and, similar to my parents and me, wants my diabetes to be in good control. But, this concern can sometimes turn him into feeling more like a parent than a spouse. Your child will want to discuss this with their significant other, and determine what, if any, accountability they want. (This can also be an issue with close friends, but mostly occurs with significant others due to the closer relationship.)

Because Type 1 diabetes is so exhausting and relentless, having a really good support system is important. I, unfortunately, know many people who have partners who guilt-trip them about all the costs and can't be bothered to help in any way. I'm totally self-sufficient now, but I also know from experience that Aaron won't hesitate to get me a regular soda if I go low while we're out and about, for example.

Your child needs to know how important it is to find their own support system—a few close friends, a group through work or church, or a significant other—who will be a source of encouragement and support. They need to feel comfortable sharing their diabetes struggles, and ask others for help when needed.

Pregnancy

If you have a daughter who has Type 1 diabetes, she may want to have children of her own someday. As of the writing of this book, I have not had children, but my mother did talk to me about pregnancy when I was in high school. While I was not planning on having children at that age, she talked to me—warned me—about the importance of good blood sugar control before and during pregnancy.

Your child needs to know how important it is to find their own support system.

Jessica Moritz, who has had diabetes for 22 years and has one daughter, said that it's important to remember that your daughter knows her body and how her body behaves with diabetes. Your daughter has a voice—a very important voice—and shouldn't ever let anyone override her own instinct.

Contrary to what you might have read online or seen in movies like *Steel Magnolias,* many women can safely have children of their own. It's more than possible, but it does take work and extra care. Morning sickness or a general inability to keep food down causes low blood sugars, and intense cravings for weird food can cause high blood sugars, but what's most important is that your daughter's blood sugars don't stay there. One of the most important details is to consistently maintain a healthy blood sugar level. According to the American Diabetes Association, women with poorly controlled blood sugars put themselves and their babies at risk for more complications.

If possible, before your daughter becomes pregnant, she should talk with her endocrinologist. This is important so that her endocrinologist can evaluate the current state of her diabetes, and give her the "okay" to conceive. Your daughter will also want to find an obstetrician who has experience with pregnancies and mothers who have Type 1 diabetes.

Diabetes in the Workplace

My own experience, and talking with many other diabetics, shows it is more than possible to have a full-time job with minimal disruptions from diabetes. After college, I worked at four different organizations and never had a major issue at work. Ironically, I now work for myself, and there have been a handful of times when I've had a low blood sugar happen during a client phone call—luckily nothing too serious, but still a bit problematic. (I've also had a few low blood sugars while writing this book!)

I recommend having a bin or drawer at work for supplies (extra test strips, extra pump supplies, glucose tabs, hard candies, packets of honey, granola bars, etc.). You never know when the vending machine at work will break down, and your child won't want to be left stranded without treatment options. I even recommend bringing a small juice or some hard candies into long meetings, so that they can treat a low blood sugar without having to leave.

Just as they did with classmates and friends, your child will one day need to tell their colleagues and bosses about their diabetes. It's not something they have to disclose during an interview. In fact, an employer cannot legally ask applicants if they have diabetes, according to the Americans with Disabilities Act (ADA).

While most employers are considerate of the needs of those who have diabetes at work, there's always the chance that your child may have difficulties with the way their employer responds to their diabetes. This could mean problems with how often they have low blood sugars, problems with the noise of their devices, or even problems with having a diabetic alert dog. But, they are protected by the ADA in a few different ways.

Accommodations

If your child has a job with physical activity or limited breaks during work hours, their employer is required to provide reasonable accommodations, something they can talk to the HR department or representative about. According to the ADA, examples of reasonable accommodations may include privacy to check their blood sugar, breaks for snacks, or slight changes to shift times. Their employer is not required to oblige to every accommodation request, especially if it's one that is difficult to accommodate or expensive.

Privacy

A potential employer cannot ask your child if they have diabetes during an interview, nor are they required to disclose it. But after making a job offer, an employer may ask questions about their health and can even require a medical exam, as long as all applicants for the same type of job are asked the same questions and required to get an exam.

Your child may think that it's not necessary to tell their coworkers or their boss because they are an adult and have things under control. Informing some of their colleagues about their diabetes is a smart idea to protect themselves, though. Sudden spikes or blood sugar drops can happen to anyone, at any time. If their blood sugar drops while they're at work, they could pass out or make an error in their work.

Your child could start with one person and slowly tell others as they become more comfortable. This will also depend on the size of their company or department. If they're one of 100, it may make sense to only tell their closest friends at work. But, if they work on a small team of seven every day, it might make the most sense to tell everyone.

What's important to remember is that your child is in control of who they tell and when. It's not legal for their boss to disclose their diagnosis to their coworkers without your child's consent. According to the ADA, their boss is only allowed to disclose your child's diagnosis to supervisors who need medical information in order to provide any necessary accommodations.

Ellie Hook, whom I've mentioned in previous chapters, shared that she's always approached telling her coworkers about her diabetes as it comes up naturally. Often, people in the office will notice her checking her blood sugar or taking insulin, which starts the conversation.

Medical Leave

As you know, you can't drive while your blood sugar is low. So, going low right as your child needs to leave for work can be quite problematic. Even worse, your child may end up in the hospital with DKA and need to miss a few days of work.

Depending on your child's employer, they could be protected by the Family and Medical Leave Act (FMLA). According to the U.S. Department of Labor, FMLA allows eligible employees to take up to 12 workweeks of unpaid, job-protected leave for certain family and medical reasons, including serious health problems that makes the employee unable to perform the essential functions of his or her job.

But, if your child's employer has a reasonable belief that they may be unable to perform their job, the employer may ask for a note from their doctor. For example, if your child needs to adjust their hours because of the current state of your diabetes, their employer may ask them to provide a doctor's note indicating there are limits on how many hours a day they can work.

Alert Dogs

Lauren Burke, whom you met in Chapter 3 and who has a diabetic alert dog, was very open at work from the beginning about her Type 1 diabetes and her dog. She even gave a presentation to everyone on her first day at a new job, explaining diabetes, her alert dog, Ricki, and how they should behave around Ricki. Lauren shared that her coworkers really struggled with the "no touch, no talk, no eye contact" rule, but eventually they got it.

When Lauren moved to another job, she ran into some problems. The building management company told Lauren she couldn't have Ricki in most parts of the building--which is illegal. To make matters worse, they also said she could only relieve Ricki in a particular spot outside. It's important to know your rights, and the ADA allows an alert dog to accompany its owner into all public places, including restaurants, stores, and schools.

Action Steps
1. When age appropriate, talk to your child about the impact of drinking alcohol as a Type 1 diabetic.
2. Before your child goes to college, consider having a conversation with them about handling their diabetes while at college and at work.

Conclusion

...

So, now what? What do you do next?

Focus on what can, or does, go right. So much of our time as individuals with Type 1 diabe-

Focus on what can, or does, go right.

tes is already spent thinking about what can wrong, or listening to our doctors lecture us about what we're doing wrong. Individuals with Type 1 diabetes need an advocate, an ally, and a cheerleader.

While I do still struggle with guilt sometimes, as I mentioned previously, I understand as an adult that while it was sometimes a challenge for others, it wasn't a burden because they loved me. My hope, in sharing some of these experiences, is that you can work to prevent the guilt from building up in your child.

Take it a day at a time. That may sound cliche, but it's some of the best advice when dealing with diabetes. As I mentioned before, there are patterns you may notice in your child, but doing the same thing day after day can still yield different results. Your child may have weeks when their sugars are all over the place, which can be overwhelming and frustrating. So, focus on today.

You feel overwhelmed right now and might be wondering, *How will I figure out the next 10 or 20 years?* It will get easier. It may not ever be easy, but it will get easier. Don't give in. My father has mentioned to me that being a parent of a child with Type 1 diabetes might be one of the hardest things he's done as a parent. You might feel like you are losing the battle, like you are overwhelmed, like you just can't keep it up. I mentioned that your child might need to see a counselor at some point, but you may need to also. Work through your emotions, instead of suppressing your feelings.

If you have a problem or a question, call someone and get the answer. Never feel like you are a bother to anyone; this is your child's life. You know your child's life is the most important thing to you. So if you need help, call as many doctors, nurses, help lines, or other parents with the same issues as you need to until you get a satisfactory answer. My dad sometimes joked that the staff at the doctor's office was probably looking at the caller ID and playing rock, paper, scissors to see who got to answer his and my mom's next question.

Finding a community of other parents who have children with Type 1 diabetes may be a great source of insight and comfort. If there is not a camp in your area, there are online communities that could be a good option. There are numerous Facebook groups for people with Type 1 diabetes, as well as parents of diabetics, those who follow certain meal plans, or just general support groups.

Lastly, know that your child will make it through this and be better for it. I hate math, but I can calculate the carbs in almost any food at the drop of a hat, in my head. I'm resilient and adapt to change fairly easy. Who knew that a three-year-old, diagnosed with Type 1 diabetes 24 years ago, would be writing this book for you to read to help you navigate life with your child's diabetes?

What might your child be doing 20 years from now to impact others?

Resources

For these resources and many more, visit https://www.the-type1life.com.

American Diabetes Association
http://www.diabetes.org/

Juvenile Diabetes Research Foundation (JDRF)
http://www.jdrf.org/

Beyond Type 1
https://beyondtype1.org/

Diabetes Daily
https://www.diabetesdaily.com/

T1 Everyday Magic
https://www.t1everydaymagic.com

Diabetes Burnout: What to Do When You Can't Take it Anymore
by William Polonsky

Dr. Bernstein's Diabetes Solution: A Complete Guide to Achieving Normal Blood Sugars
By Richard K. Bernstein, http://www.diabetes-book.com/

Taking Diabetes to School
by Kim Gosselin

MySugr: Diabetes Tracker Log
https://mysugr.com/

MyFitnessPal
http://www.myfitnesspal.com/

CalorieKing
http://www.calorieking.com/

Sugarmate
https://sugarmate.io/

Diabits
https://www.diabits.com

Glossary

504 plan: According to Understood.org, a blueprint for how the school will provide supports and remove barriers for a student with a disability, so the student has equal access to the general education curriculum.

A1C: According to the American Diabetes Association, a test that gives you a picture of your average blood glucose (blood sugar) control for the past two to three months.

Carbohydrates: According to Merriam-Webster.com, a substance (as a starch or sugar) that is rich in energy and is made up of carbon, hydrogen, and oxygen. *(These are one of the things your child takes insulin for.)*

Continuous Glucose Monitor (CGM): According to Dexcom.com, an FDA-approved device that provides continuous insight into glucose levels throughout the day and night. The device displays information about glucose direction and speed providing users additional information to help with their diabetes management.

Diabulimia: According to the National Eating Disorders Association, the reduction of insulin intake by Type 1 diabetics in an effort to lose weight.

Endocrinology: According to Merriam-Webster.com, a branch of medicine concerned with the structure, function, and disorders of the endocrine glands. *(You will visit your child's endocrinologist every few months to make adjustments to their diabetes care.)*

Glucagon: According to Merriam-Webster.com, a protein hormone that is produced especially by the islets of Langerhans and that promotes an increase in the sugar content of the blood by increasing the rate of glycogen breakdown in the liver. *(A glucagon kit should be kept on hand in case of severe hypoglycemia.)*

Glucose tabs: According to WebMD.com, chewable sugar tablets used by people with diabetes to raise their blood sugar quickly when it drops dangerously low, a condition known as hypoglycemia.

Glucometer: According to the FDA, a test system for use at home to measure the amount of sugar (glucose) in your blood. *(Also referred to as just a "meter," a glucometer should be kept near your child at all times, so they can check their blood sugar at a moment's notice.)*

Hypoglycemia: According to Merriam-Webster.com, an abnormal decrease of sugar in the blood. *(Hypoglycemia is also referred to as a "low blood sugar.")*

Hyperglycemia: According to Merriam-Webster.com, an excess of sugar in the blood. *(Hyperglycemia is also referred to as a "high blood sugar.")*

IEP (individualized education program): According to Understood.org, a document that spells out your child's learning needs, the services the school will provide, and how progress will be measured. *(Students may get a 504 plan instead of an IEP.)*

Ketones: According to the American Diabetes Association, a chemical produced when there is a shortage of insulin in the blood and the body breaks down body fat for energy.

About the Author

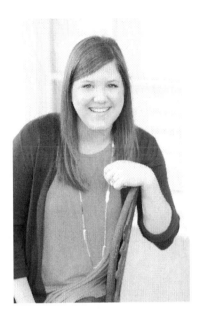

Jessica Freeman is a Type 1 diabetes advocate, has been living with Type 1 diabetes for 26 years, and is the author of *The Type 1 Life for Adults*. Jessica is also the owner of Jess Creatives, an award-winning graphic and web design company. Jessica lives in Atlanta, Georgia, with her husband, Aaron, and their cocker spaniel, Morgan Freeman.